A Guide to
Cast Care

By Kenneth Wright
In consultation with members of the NAOT (National Association of Orthopedic Technologists), and the CSOT (Canadian Society of Orthopedic Technologists), Brian Abdul, Roberta Charlesworth, Sean Conkle, Michael Gill, Cynthia Henderson and Dion Maxwell.

Also consulted, NAON (National Association of Orthopedic Nurses), CONA (Canadian Association of Orthopedic Nurses), and PAPE (Physician's Association for Patient Education).

Cast Care self help patient manual

ISBN # 1 55040-208-0

1022007

1

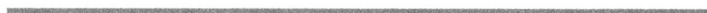

CONTACTS

Fill these in for easy reference

Doctor's name ....

         Office phone...

         Emergency phone ....

Hospital ....

         General phone.......................................

         Emergency Department phone ....

Registered Orthopedic
Technologist's name ....

Neighbors who can help you

         Name...

         Phone..

         Name ....

         Phone..

         Name ....

         Phone..

Taxi phone ....

Ambulance phone ....

CONTENTS

ORTHOPEDIC HEALTH CARE
PROFESSIONAL SPECIALISTS

Orthopedic Surgeons
These specialist surgeons are the team leaders for all musculoskeletal health conditions of patients, and through research, innovation, practice and association, advance the medical science of orthopedics.
For more information visit:
www.aaos.org

Orthopedic Technologists
A certified trained assistant to the orthopedic surgeon, usually working in a fracture clinic or operating suite. Their main duties include: applies and removes casts, fits and adjusts canes, crutches and walkers, plans and implements traction procedures, applies braces and prosthetics, fabricates and applies splints and bandages, and educates patients.
For more information visit:
(Canada) www.pappin.com/csot
Canadian Society of Orthopedic Technologists.

(US) www.naot.org
National Association of Orthopedic Technologists

Orthopedic Nurses
These qualified nurses specialize in orthopedics and ensure all aspects of the orthopedic patient are addressed to ensure a successful and comprehensive healing is achieved.
For more information visit:
(Canada) www.cona-nurse.org
Canadian Association of Orthopedic Nurses

(US) www.orthonurse.org
National Association of Orthopedic Nurses

Orthopedic Physician Assistants
These orthopedic certified individuals enhance the quality of medical treatment of orthopedic patients by providing skilled professional and mid – level medical physician extenders to Orthopedic Surgeons.
For more information visit:
www.asopa.org
American Association of Orthopedic Physicians Assistants

INTRODUCTION

You are probably reading this book because you or a loved one is going to be wearing a cast for the next few weeks. If you had a choice you would probably prefer to read a good novel or maybe watch TV. With this in mind, this book has been written in a note-form way – lots of headings so that you can quickly reference what you need to know.

Look upon the cast as a new body part. It goes with you all the time, taking part in all your activities, often making you a focal point of the people around you, not to mention encouraging your friends to sign the cast or write a wisecrack on it.

Rest assured, though, casts have been around for many centuries so you can be confident of the medical soundness of such a treatment. Even Hippocrates in the fourth century B.C. was reported to have used a mixture of gum and flour dough to mend a variety of injuries. The practice did not spread to Europe until the 19th century; there is a record of Napoleon's surgeon using a bandage that was made from a complicated mixture which even included wine and egg whites! These early casts took a long time to set and people had to sit or lie down without moving for days.

Eventually "plaster of Paris" arrived (named after plaster deposits found near the French capital) which is historically closest to modern day casts. It was an awkward procedure involving plaster moulds being attached to a complicated array of bandages. However, the modern day plaster casts have proven to be extremely successful and highly practical for many years.

It will take some time to adjust to your cast. Naturally, during the first few days you will be constantly aware of its presence. To help become accustomed to it, take it easy and do activities slower than normal. In time you will adjust to the temporary physical limitations and may be pleasantly surprised at how well you actually cope with your normal day to day activities. Remember though that your injury takes time to heal and always be cautious in your activities to avoid further complications.

Each year there are estimated to be 250,000 casts worn in Canada for fractures and sprains, so you are definitely not alone. Invest in a little time to read this book or reference parts of the book when you need specific information. The benefit to you, wearing the cast , or to your caregiver or family member, is that with understanding you can avoid complications, comply to the advice of your health care practitioner and achieve timely, successful healing.

THE OUTSTANDING FEATURES OF PLASTER CASTS ARE:

1. They harden quickly

2. They are easy to apply

3. They are durable and strong

There are a variety of types of casts today, each type offering certain advantages. Your medical team will decide which one is best for you.

All casts are strong and protective and are constructed to keep your injury immobile so that it can heal properly. Although wearing a cast can be annoying and inconvenient, it will keep the injured bones, ligaments and muscles from moving so they can heal as naturally and strongly as is possible.

The purpose of this book is to help you understand the role your cast plays in the healing process. More importantly, there is information on how you can help yourself during this often trying time and how you can get the most benefit from your cast by managing and caring for this new "body part".

One of the most important sections within this book is "WARNING SIGNS—WHEN TO CALL YOUR DOCTOR OR FRACTURE CLINIC." Sometimes there can be problems with wearing a cast that can slow down the healing process and cause other problems. If you experience any of these Warning Signs (pg. 63) you must never be afraid or reluctant to call your doctor or return to the hospital for help. You and the medical staff are all part of a winning team, who want you to get back to your normal quality of life, just as soon as possible.

All technical terms are explained throughout the book and there are many specific headings to help you reference information.

WHY DOES THE DOCTOR APPLY A CAST?

The introduction has explained what a cast does; the four most common reasons for applying a cast in order of magnitude are:

1. To keep the ends of a broken bone (fracture) together so they can heal correctly.

2. To keep severely strained muscles and ligaments together so they can heal in an optimum fashion.

3. To keep a body part from moving after surgery or an amputation.

4. To correct a deformity such as a club foot or a hip displacement.

THE MEDICAL TEAM THAT CAN HELP YOU

The Physician/Surgeon
You will see a physician/surgeon at an office, in a hospital's emergency department, or in a fracture clinic. The physician/surgeon will be involved in diagnosis, evaluation of your injury and the healing process.

The X–ray Department
Having an X-ray is necessary to determine the extent of the injury. After your injury has been casted, you may have x–rays while the cast is still in place, to evaluate the healing procress

The Registered Orthopedic Technologist
These professionals in the hospital will be involved with initially assessing your injury and sending you to the x-ray department.
The Registered Orthopedic Technologist applies the cast to your limb, and is extremely skilled in ensuring it is applied effectively to ensure proper healing.

Physical Therapists/Physiotherapists

These people are experts in helping your muscles and bones get back to the same condition prior to the injury.

Other medical personnel

You may be treated in another facility or clinic that is not a fracture clinic. Other qualified people that can treat you may include: a family practitioner, an orthopedic nurse, an orthopedic physician's assistant or a nurse practitioner.

The Pharmacist and home care store

You may have to obtain medication, skin care products, crutches, slings and other products to help in the healing process and to provide comfort to you when you are casted. Pharmacists and home care store personnel are also trained in counselling and providing all sorts of information.

Questions you may want to ask the medical team

HOW BROKEN BONES HEAL

The minute you break a bone it starts the healing process immediately. Below are the ABCs of bone healing:

A. Blood collects at the "break" site

B one is actually a living tissue containing blood vessels which bleeds when your bone fractures along with other nearby tissues. Blood then collects around the broken bone ends, forming a sticky, jelly-like mass which is called a "clot."

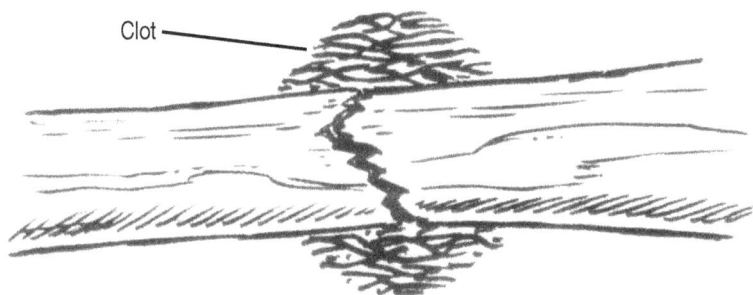

Clot ——

B. New cells enter the clot

Healing starts when new cells or living parts called "osteoclasts" and "osteoblasts" invade this clot and produce a network of fibers that begin to bind the tissues together. More specifically, the osteoclasts start dissolving the jagged edges of the bone ends. The osteoblasts start the rebuilding process by joining the various ends of the broken bones. With this process you can understand the importance of having the broken bone ends as close together as possible, to help the efficiency of the healing process.

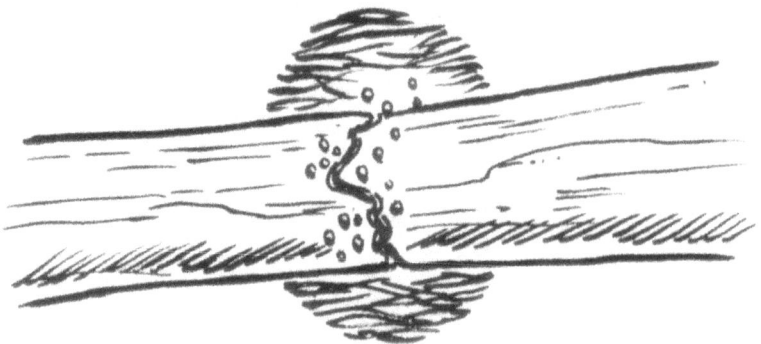

C. New bone forms

On average 6 to 10 days after the break, the mesh of cells bridging the broken bones becomes a young bony mass called a "callus" which will eventually harden to form new bone. But for now, this new bone is spongy, weak and fragile. Any abrupt motion can split it and thereby slow down the healing process. That's why the cast is very important at this stage, to keep the broken bone from moving while it is healing.

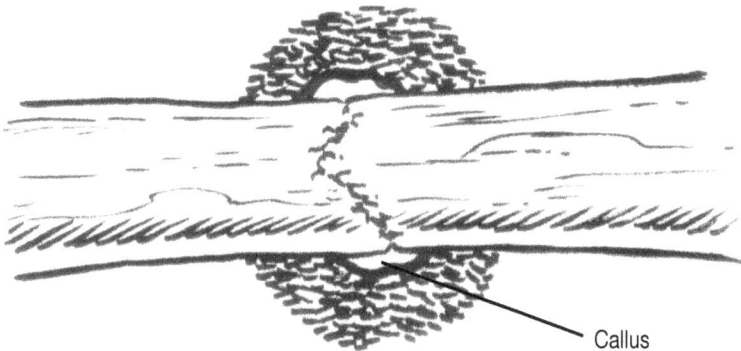

Callus

D. Bone hardens

O n average 3 to 10 weeks after the break, newly–formed blood vessels start bringing calcium to the injured area to harden the new bone tissue. This process is called "ossification" and when the process is complete, the broken bone is said to be "officially" healed and the cast is removed.

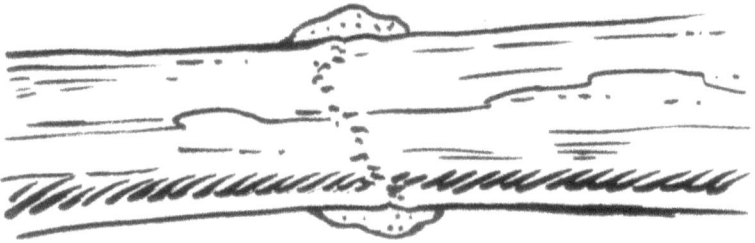

E. Continued healing to become a normal strong bone

It may take a year before the bone is healed to the point where it is as strong as it was before the break. With time and proper exercise after the cast is removed, the bone will mature and become strong. In most cases your bone will be "as good as new."

It is worth understanding that everybody is different in how well or how quickly our bones heal. The younger you are (say up to the age of 20), the faster the healing process. Older people usually have more fragile bones and are less able to take the stress and demands of movement. However, no matter how old you are, your body has an amazing ability to heal.

AVERAGE HEALING TIME FOR FRACTURES	
Bone	Number of Weeks
Collar Bone	6
Upper arm:	
Neck	6
Shaft	12
Forearm:	
Both bones	6-12
One bone	6
Hand:	4-6
Finger:	3
Hip:	12
Upper leg:	
Femur	8-12
Lower leg (fibula):	
Plateau	6-8
Shaft	12-24
Ankle	6-8
Heel:	8-12
Foot:	6-8
Toe:	3

KID'S BONES

A child's bones have characteristics that make the injury and the healing process somewhat different from the healing of adult bones. Until the early teens, children's bones are elastic and flexible. In fact, children's bones are made mostly of cartilage. As the child matures, this cartilage is replaced by the more rigid tissue, called bone.

The "green twig" comparison

When a child injures a bone, instead of breaking, because of inherent flexibility, the bone just bends or partially breaks, like the green twigs of a tree. In fact, a fracture of a child's bone is commonly called a "green stick" fracture.

Another interesting fact about children's bones is that their broken bones will often remodel themselves naturally. Just like the "green twig," the bone can become straight and tall again all on its own. Sometimes a doctor may not find it necessary to perfectly align a child's broken bone because it will remodel itself into a perfectly straight bone again in just a couple of years.

Growth plates

To allow for bone growth, children's bones have a number of fragile growth centers or plates which are located on the ends of long bones. These plates are responsible for bone growth. As the child grows older, the growth plates close and subsequently bones stop growing. However, these plates are inherently weak and can become dislodged when a bone is injured. An injury to these bone plates is common in children and can sometimes cause an arm or leg to be marginally shorter than the other arm or leg. The difference though is usually not noticeable.

Discuss your concerns with the Orthopedic Surgeon or Family Doctor.

YOUR CHOICE OF AVAILABLE CASTS

There are four different types of casts your health care practitioner may apply:

- Plaster
- Synthetic fiberglass
- Synthetic non-fiberglass material
- Cast Liner Waterproof Cast

You will see these types all in rolls and once applied to your injury, the material hardens quite quickly to form the cast. All four types of casts keep broken bones and surrounding tissue rigidly immobile. Synthetic casts also have the property of enabling X–rays to be taken if needed, so that the physician can see how well the healing process is taking place. Although all four types provide similar medical benefits, there are advantages and disadvantages to each type. You will be caring for your cast, so you should review the differences as follows:

1. Plaster cast

This cast consists of open–weave cotton rolls or strips impregnated with dry calcium sulfate (a chalky white powder made from gypsum crystals.)

Advantages
- It's easy to mold.
- It rarely causes skin irritations or an allergic reaction.
- Plaster cast material is inexpensive.

Disadvantages
- It's messy to apply.
- It's heavy and bulky, which can cause problems for children and the elderly.
- It's easily weakened by moisture.
- It dries more slowly than the other two types of casts.
- Not radiolucent—the cast has to be removed for X-rays to be taken and then reapplied.

2. Synthetic Fiberglass casts

This cast is formed from open–weave fiberglass tape impregnated with a chemical substance called polyurethane resin.

Advantages
- It is both lightweight and durable.
- It is porous, therefore it allows the skin to breathe.
- Resists weakening from moisture.
- After initial application, this cast dries quickly, within 4 to 5 minutes: it can bear body weight 20 minutes after its application.
- Less chance of a breakdown.
- Radiolucent—X-rays can be taken without removing the cast.

Disadvantages
- If not molded properly, edges can be abrasive.
- There are different molding techniques compared to plaster.
- Possibly not covered by health care plan.

3. Synthetic non-fiber casts

This cast consists of polyester and cotton open-weave tape impregnated with water-activated polyurethane.

Advantages
This cast dries in 7 minutes and it can bear body weight after 20 minutes.
- It is both lightweight and durable.
- It is porous, thereby reducing itching.
- It conforms well to body contours.
- It is radiolucent—allowing X-rays to be taken without removing the cast.

Disadvantages
- There are different molding techniques compared to plaster.
- Possibly not covered by health care plan.

4. Waterproof Casts

GORE® PROCEL® Cast Liner is a waterproof, breathable, washable cast padding that replaces standard cotton or synthetic padding underneath a fiberglass cast. Traditional cast padding absorbs and retains moisture, which often leads to skin break down and the proliferation of bacterial growth and odor. With GORE® PROCEL® Cast Liner, patients have the ability to rinse dead skin and bacteria out of the cast, and maintain their daily lifestyle activities – bathe, shower, exercise swim, etc. GORE® PROCEL® Cast Liner may also reduce the incidence of unscheduled cast changes.

Advantages
GORE® PROCEL® Cast Liner is breathable, with typical drying times under 1 hour after getting your cast wet.
GORE's® PROCEL® Cast Liner allows for routine washing and bathing, reducing the amount of odor and itching. Good skin health is maintained while wearing a cast.
GORE's® PROCEL® cast liner allows patients to maintain their normal lifestyle without worrying about getting their casts wet.
GORE® PROCEL® Cast Liner is reimbursable under most health insurance plans.

Disadvantages
GORE® PROCEL® Cast Liner may not be suitable for all casts. GORE® PROCEL® Cast Liner is not intended for use over open wounds and/or fractures. Your Physician can reference the GORE® PROCEL® Cast Liner "Instructions for Use" to determine the proper indications for PROCEL®.

MAKING SURE THE CAST DRIES PROPERLY

After your cast has been applied, it is important for it to dry thoroughly and evenly. Initially, the wet cast will feel heavy and warm, but with time, it will get lighter as the moisture evaporates from the cast. Skin problems can arise if your cast is not dried thoroughly, so do not underestimate this important aspect.

Here are some tips to ensure success:

1. Keep excess moisture away from the cast

When you elevate the cast on pillows, make sure the pillows have rubber or plastic covers under the pillow case. Use a thin towel placed between the cast and the pillows to absorb the moisture. Never place a wet cast directly onto plastic.

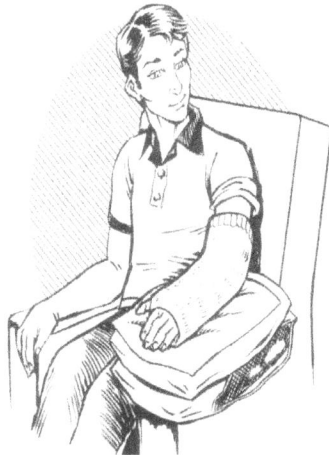

2. Tips to speed up drying time

Keep the cast exposed to air, especially plaster casts, which take much longer to dry, sometimes as long as 48 hours. Drying a plaster cast in less time makes it more comfortable and manageable sooner.

3. Ensure even drying

Change your position on pillows every 2 hours, using the palms of your hands instead of your finger tips. Your palms have a larger surface area and can prevent any indents made on the cast by your fingers.

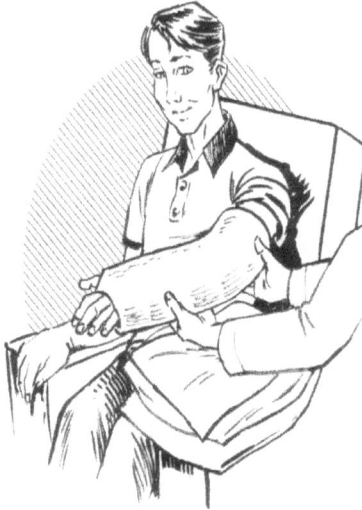

4. Prevent bumps inside the cast

To avoid creating bumps inside the cast, do not poke at the cast, particularly if the cast has not completely dried. These bumps can cause serious skin irritations or sores during the time you are wearing your cast.

CAST CARE MANAGEMENT TIPS

Follow your health care practitioner's instructions carefully, especially regarding physical activity.

1. Protect your cast

Make sure you do not knock or rest your cast against any hard surface. Protect the foot of a leg cast from scrapes, breakage or dirt.

Try this:

Wear a big sock over the cast to keep toes warm and cast clean. Always wear a cast boot if walking is allowed. Place a carpet square over the bottom of the cast. Cut a V-shape at the back, so that the carpet fits around the heel when you bring it toward the ankle. Then hold the carpet in place with a large sock or slipper sock. Finally, extend the carpet out beyond the toes a little and this will help prevent toes from being bumped or stubbed.

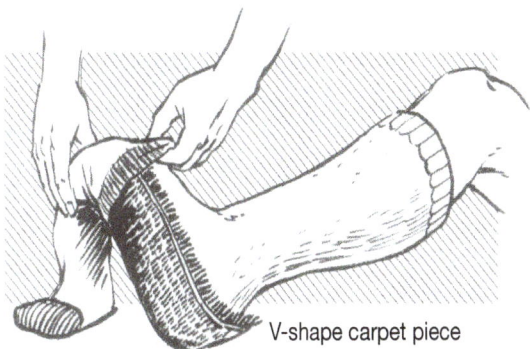

V-shape carpet piece

2. Prevent snags

To keep an arm cast from snagging clothing and furniture, make a cast cover from an old nylon stocking. Cut the stocking's toe off and cut a hole in the heel. Then pull the stocking over the cast to cover it. Extend your fingers through the cut-off toe end and poke your thumb through the hole you cut in the heel. Trim the other end of the stocking to about 1½" longer than the cast. Finally, tuck the ends of the stocking under the cast's edges.

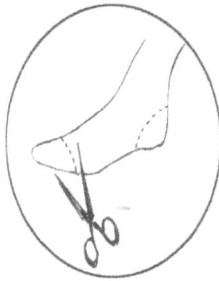

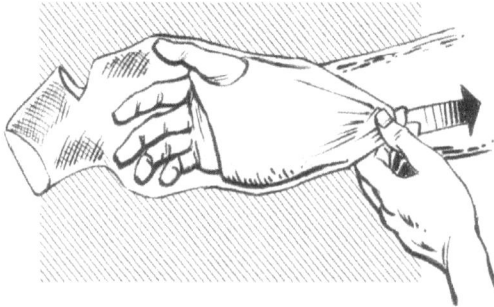

3. Keep your cast dry

Keep your cast dry while bathing, showering or swimming. How? Wrap cast in a towel and wrap tightly with two plastic bags or purchase a cast protector. If unsure, keep the affected limb out of the bathtub/shower.

A. Plaster cast precautions

It is vital that you do not let a plaster cast get wet. Moisture will weaken or destroy it. If you accidently get the cast wet by walking in the rain or whatever, contact your fracture clinic. When plaster gets wet, it becomes permanently compromised.

B. Fiberglass or synthetic cast precautions

First and foremost to know, check with your physician or orthopedic technologist if you may bathe, shower or swim with the cast on. If you have an unstable fracture or there is an open wound, you should use the same advice listed under plaster cast precautions.

C. Caring for your Cast when using GORE® PROCEL® Cast Liner

GORE® PROCEL® Cast Liner may be utilized as padding under most extremity fracture casts. It should not be applied to open wounds and/or fractures. Under your Physician's guidance, patients may bathe, shower, swim and undergo hydrotherapy while wearing their cast. Care should be taken to thoroughly rinse underneath the cast padding with clean water to remove residual soap, shampoo, chlorine, salt, dirt or other substances. Routing washing followed by thorough rinsing inside the cast will reduce odor, irritation, and improve overall skin hygiene of the cast area. No special drying procedures are required after getting the cast wet. Drying times will vary depending upon environmental conditions. However, the majority of casts will completely dry after 1 hour. The use of a blower or hair dryer is not recommended. In addition, baby powder, talc powder, lotions and other oils should not be applied under the cast padding. You should consult the GORE® PROCEL® Cast Liner patient brochure for complete cast care information.

4. Avoid scratching under your cast

Although itching is a nuisance and irritating try to avoid this - time usually solves the problem. Breaking the skin under the cast can cause serious problems like an infection.

Especially avoid using coat hangers or any sharp objects to scratch the itch; these objects can really cause damage. Also avoid stuffing toilet paper or cotton under the cast's edges. To relieve the itching try sprinkling baby powder into the end of your cast. Another effective technique can be the use of a hand held blow dryer set at "cool" and aimed at the problem area. Minimize perspiration.

5. Prevent swelling

Elevate your cast. Especially during the first few days after your cast is applied. The aim is to have your cast above your heart. This will prevent harmful swelling by allowing the blood fluids that have collected near the injury to drain

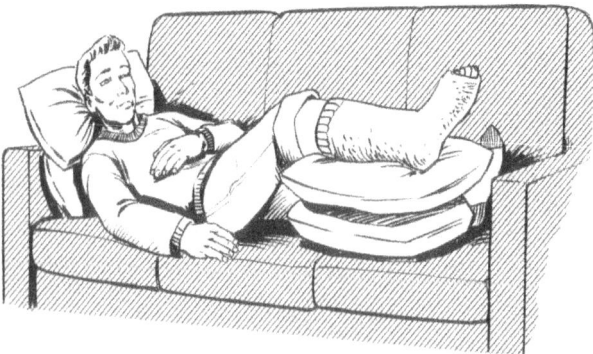

"downhill." Obviously, there will be some swelling, which is normal, but excessive swelling should be avoided. Compare your casted arm or leg with the other one to evaluate how much swelling you have. Your physician will tell you how long and how often your cast should be elevated.

6. Check for changes in sensation, movement or circulation
Several times a day check for sensations by touching the areas above and below the cast. Here are the pointers to look for:

1. Feeling of numbness.
2. Tingling feeling.
3. Pain. (excessive)
4. Unable to wiggle fingers or toes.
5. Pain when wiggling fingers or toes.
6. Press fingernail or large toenail of the casted limb until it turns white, then let go. If normal pink color does not return within 3 seconds then that is a warning sign.
7. If your fingers or toes are cold first try covering them. If that does not warm them then that is a warning sign.
8. Finally if any of these changes take place—contact your fracture clinic or doctor.

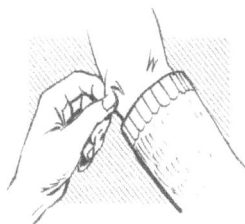

| Checking Sensation | Checking Circulation | Checking Movement |

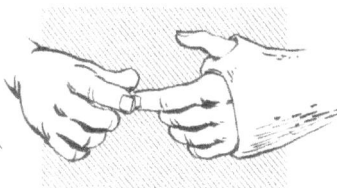

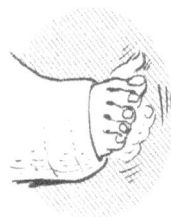

7. Sleeping with a cast

Experiment with ways to make sleeping more comfortable. Try placing pillows under and around your cast to cushion it. Wiggling is not sufficient.

8. Exercise your fingers or toes

Wiggle them back and forth. This can improve your blood circulation which is vital in getting the healing nutrients to your injury. Exercise and getting that blood pumping is the most important thing you can do to help healing. This will reduce swelling and prevent stiffness.

9. Never stuff material inside your cast

Never insert cotton, tissue or anything into the ends of the cast. The danger is that this material may work its way into the cast, which can create pressure, that could result into a medical problem such as creating a worsening sore.

10. Avoid irritation from rough cast edges

After the cast completely dries, rough edges may cause skin irritation. To smooth them, try these techniques:

For fibreglass casts simply remove the rough edges by filing the edges with a nail file to smooth them out.

For a plaster cast you can "petal" rough edges using adhesive tape or moleskin. This prevents catching the material on clothing or peeling it off accidently.

To do this, cut several 4" by 2" strips of tape or moleskin and trim the ends that will be outside the cast so that they are rounded like toenails.

Next, place the first strip, rounded end down on the outside of the cast; then tuck the straight end just inside the cast edge. Smooth the tape or moleskin with your finger to remove any creases - which can also cause irritation of the skin. Repeat this with overlap strips as needed until you have covered all the rough edges with protective "petals."

Cutting the Petals

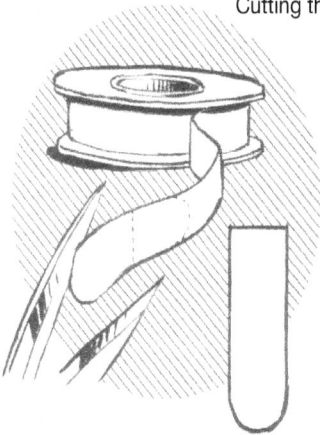

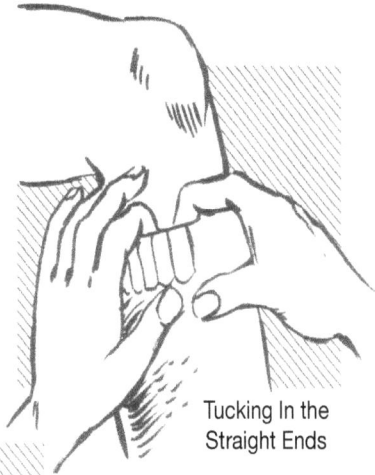

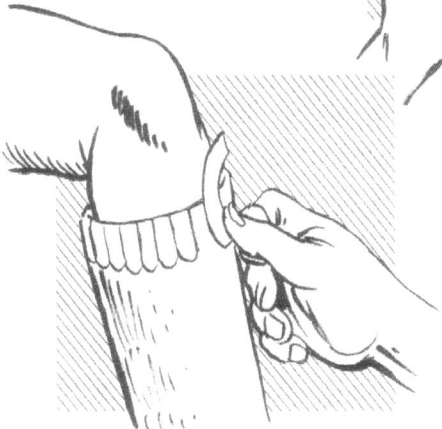

Tucking In the Straight Ends

Attaching the Petals

11. Care for your skin

You should wash the skin along the cast's edges every day using a mild soap. However, before you start you should protect the cast's edges with plastic wrap to avoid wetting it excessively. Then use a washcloth wrung out in soapy water to cleanse the skin where it meets the cast edges, and as far as you can reach inside the cast. Dry the skin thoroughly with a towel, then massage the skin at the cast edges and under them with a towel or pad saturated with rubbing alcohol. This will help toughen the skin. A final tip to prevent skin irritation, is to remove any loose plaster particles that you can reach inside the cast.

12. Check the fit of your cast

The general rule for checking to see if the fit is right is to slip two fingers into the cast. If you can fit more than two fingers inside the cast, it is too loose. If you cannot fit two fingers inside the cast, it is too tight. Remember: a loose cast can prevent proper bone alignment and a tight cast can impair your blood circulation.

13. Drainage from the cast

When a cast covers a wound, you can expect some drainage during the first 48 hours after the cast is applied. Often the drainage stains the actual cast. If this occurs it will help your health care professional if you mark the drainage site on the cast with a felt pen. Outline the stain with the pen and write the date and time on the cast.

You must notify your doctor if any of the following occur:
1. Drainage amounts increase.
2. Drainage stains the cast or bed linen bright red.
3. Drainage occurs even though the cast was not applied over a wound.
4. The odour or colour of the drainage changes.

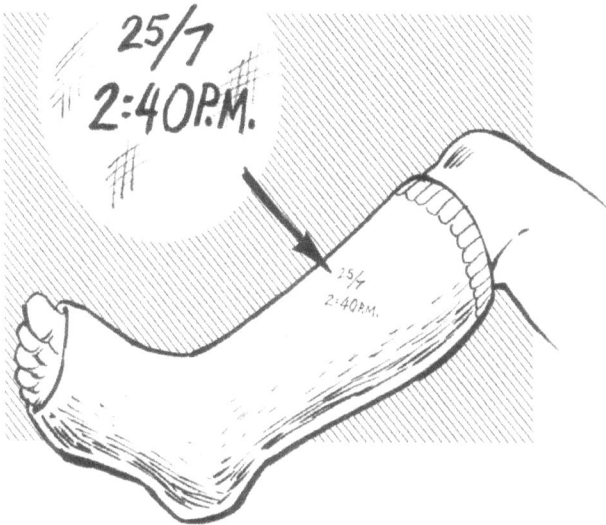

14. Using a sling for an arm cast

This may be recommended for support of an arm in a cast. Change it regularly because a soiled sling can cause irritation and possibly infection. Make sure you have professional help in applying the sling and make sure a family member or friend can position the sling correctly. Support the wrist to prevent wrist damage, knot the sling effectively, place the sling around the clothing to reduce pressure on the neck and shoulder and adjust the sling for the right angle.

See the diagrams below.

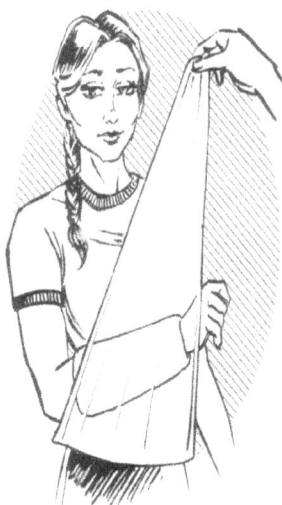

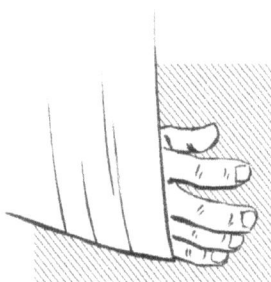

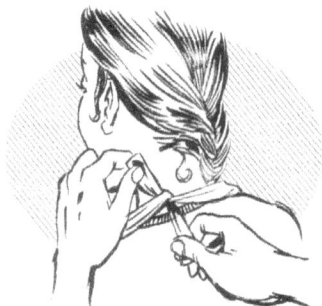

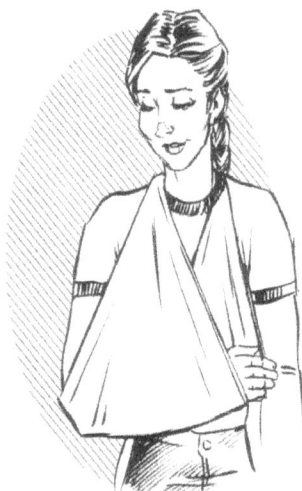

USING CRUTCHES

Pressure from your body weight when standing or walking on a casted leg can slow down the healing process of some fractures. Crutches have been designed to solve this problem by helping reduce the amount of weight you put on a casted leg or foot.

You will be instructed to walk with crutches with one of the following methods:

1. Non weight bearing:

No weight to be placed on your injured leg. This means you must always keep your casted leg off the floor.

2. Featherweight bearing:

Able to put your casted leg on the floor, just for balance.

3. Partial weight bearing:

Able to put a designated amount of weight on your casted leg as recommended by your health care practitioner.

4. Weight bearing as tolerated:

Able to take all the weight on your casted leg.

The following guidelines may help you :

1. Fitting of crutches

To ascertain the right sized crutches, stand up straight with the crutches 6" to the side of your feet. The underarm pieces of the crutches should be at about 1-1½" (roughly two finger widths) below your armpits. If the underarm pieces touch your armpits, ask to have the crutch's length adjusted. The crutch tops should not be supporting your weight; that is the job of the hand grips. You should check the placement of the handgrips. When you grasp them, make sure they are at wrist level.

2. Using crutches properly

Always use your arms, not your armpits, to support your weight. If, when you are walking with your crutches, you feel a tingling sensation or numbness in the side of your chest below your armpits, or in your upper arms, you are probably using your crutches improperly or you may just need to have the size adjusted.

Check that your crutches are in good condition.

The three most important issues are :
1. Rubber tips at the base to prevent sliding.
2. Padded underarm pieces for comfort and hand grips should be padded.
3. Check all wing nuts daily.

A. With no weight on your injured leg.

1. Positioning yourself

Stand straight, with all your weight on your uninjured leg. Relax your shoulders. Hold the foot of your injured leg off the floor, flexing your knee slightly. Balance all your weight on the crutches and position the uninjured leg and the crutches to support your weight as you lean your body slightly forward.

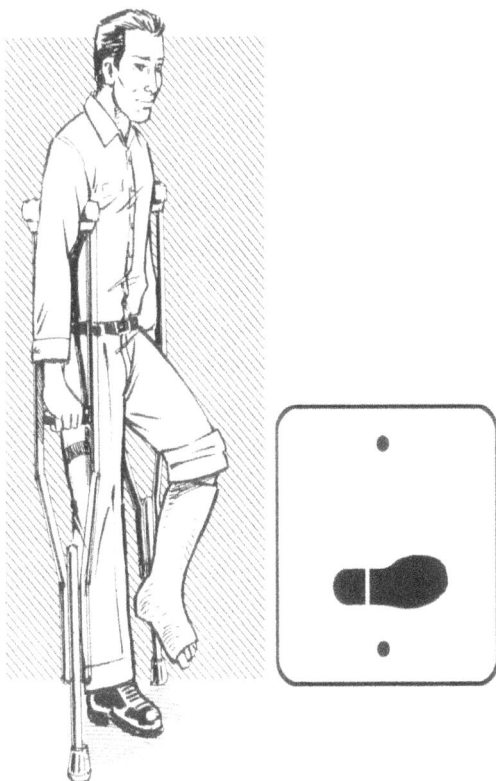

2. Shifting your weight

Shift all your weight to the uninjured leg and move the crutches forward together, swinging the injured leg along with them. Make sure you do not put any weight on the injured leg.

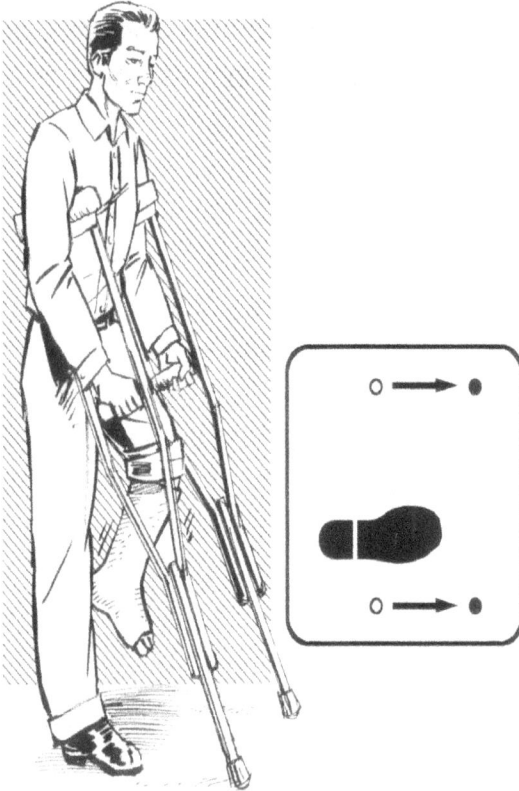

3. Moving forward

Now shift all your weight back to the crutches, swing your uninjured leg forward and again place all your weight on this leg just using the crutches to keep your balance.

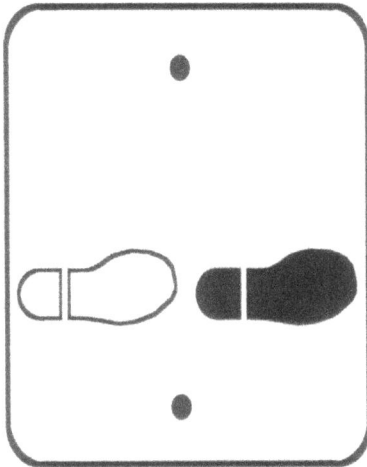

To keep walking repeat points 2 and 3 above.

B. With partial weight on your injured leg.

1. Distributing your weight

Stand straight with your shoulders relaxed and your arms slightly bent. Lean your body slightly forward distributing your weight between the crutches and your uninjured leg. You can put some weight on your injured leg.

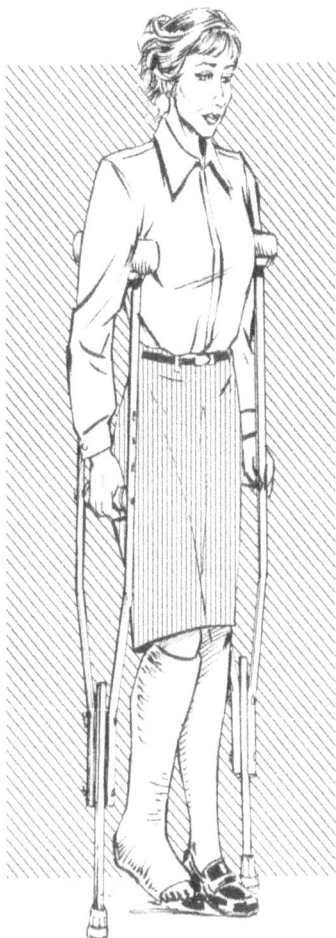

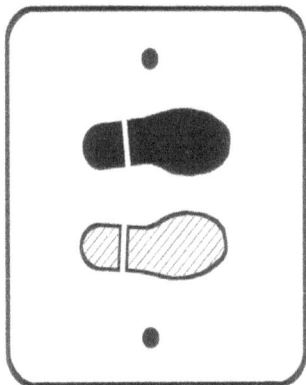

2. Moving the crutches

Move the crutches forwards then move your injured leg up to them.

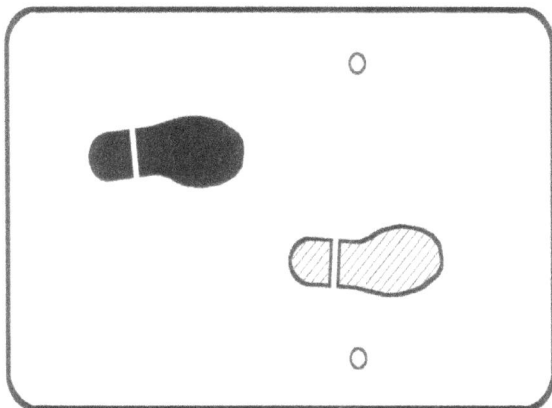

3. Moving forward

Put some weight on your injured leg as you move your uninjured leg ahead of the crutches. Continue in this manner.

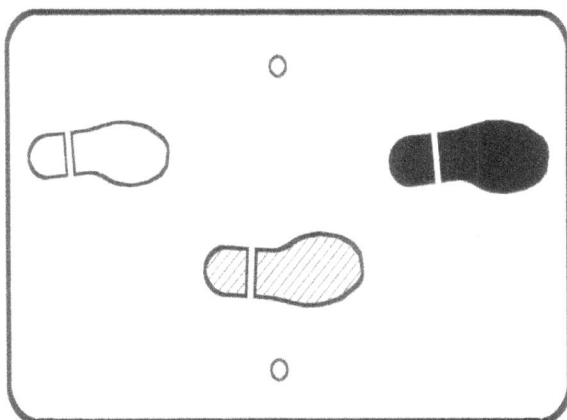

Sitting down and getting up with crutches

Sitting down

Stand with the backs of your knees against the chair's front edge. Positioning your weight on the uninjured leg, transfer both crutches to the hand on the same side as your injured leg. Then supporting most of your weight on the crutches, reach back with your other hand and grasp the chair arm, keeping your weight off your injured leg.

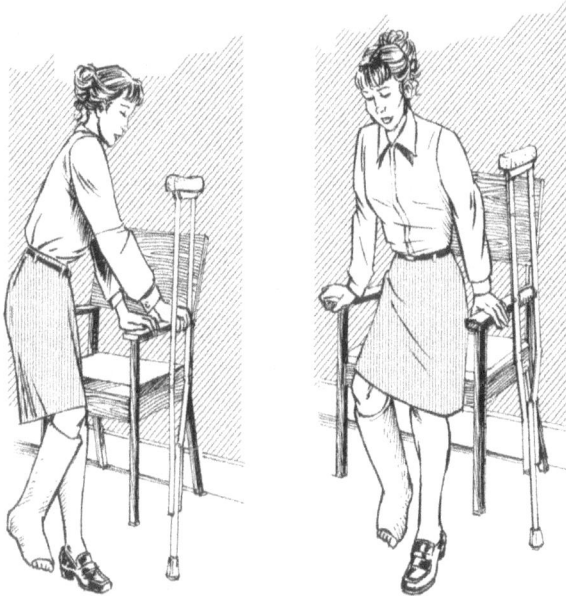

Getting up

Make sure first the chair is stable. Pivot on your uninjured leg so the back of that leg touches the chair seat. Put your other hand on the other chair arm. Support your weight with your hands. Slide forward, with your uninjured leg slightly under the chair. Grasp the chair arms and push yourself up onto the uninjured leg. Once you are standing, pivot on the uninjured leg with the hand on the same side grasping the chair arm to pick up the crutches. Then transfer one of the crutches to your uninjured leg side to start walking.

Using crutches on stairs

Positioning yourself

The banister is positioned on the left for these instructions.

Standing at the bottom of the stairs, shift both crutches to your right hand. Now grasp the banister firmly with your left hand. Using the right hand, carefully support your weight on the crutches.

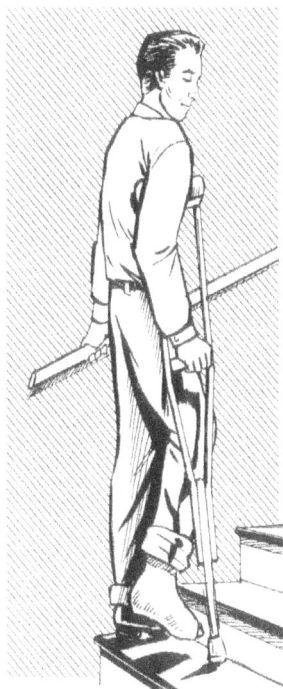

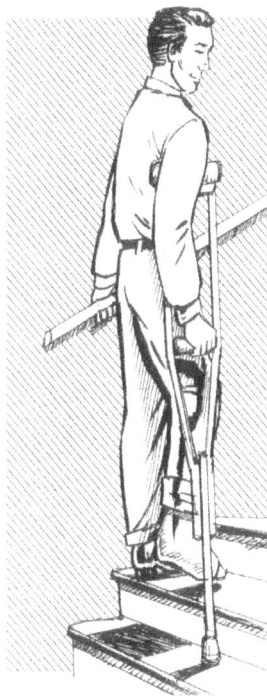

Moving up and down the stairs

Now push down on both crutches and hop onto the first step, using your uninjured leg. Support your weight on that leg as you continue to grasp the banister tightly. Then swing the crutches up onto the first step. Now hop onto the second step, using your uninjured leg. Repeat this procedure, but go slowly.

To get down the stairs, reverse these guidelines. Make sure you advance your crutches and your uninjured leg <u>first.</u>

Using only one crutch or a cane

Always use the crutch or the cane in the hand opposite to the injured leg. This will give you better support and helps you perform the normal movements of walking.

GENERAL SAFETY TIPS

| 1 | Always use your arms to support your weight. Do not rest your crutches in your armpits. The constant pressure could damage the nerves under your armpits. |

| 2 | If you feel any numbness or tingling below your armpits and fingers or in your upper arms, you are probably using the crutches incorrectly. |

| 3 | Never stand on your injured leg without your health care professional's approval. |

| 4 | Avoid wet surfaces where possible. Use smaller steps if you walk on a wet or slippery surface. |

| 5 | Scatter rugs or throw mats should be removed as they can slip and cause you to fall. |

| 6 | Wear good supporting shoes or bare feet rather than slippers. |

| 7 | Make sure your crutches are in good condition, check out the rubber tips, pads under the armpits, hand grips and wing nuts. |

EXERCISES FOR CASTED LIMBS

Depending on which of your limbs has a cast, your health care professional may recommend exercises for the non-casted joint(s) on that limb. When you exercise these joint(s), it will help keep the entire limb strong during this healing period.

Of course, you must always follow the specific instructions from your health care professional. You will probably be told to do the exercises several times a day.

Here are some common examples of exercises that can usually help you:

Exercising fingers

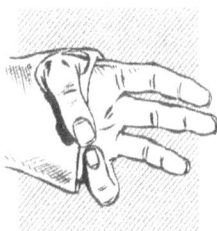

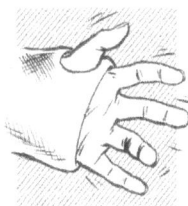

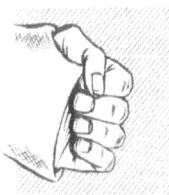

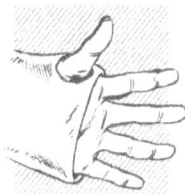

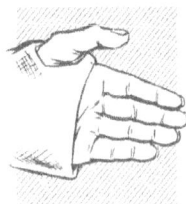

Hold up your hand and separate the fingers; then close them up. Next, hold up your hand and touch the little finger and thumb together. Finally bend all the fingers on your hands up and down, as though you were waving goodbye to someone. Bend and straighten elbow if a short arm cast is applied.

Exercising the wrist

With your forearm resting on the arm of a chair and your hand extended straight out, with your palm down, bend your wrist slowly up and down to raise and lower your hand.

Exercising the shoulder joint

With your arm straight down at your side and the palm of your hand next to your body, swing your arm out and up until it is even with your shoulder. Now bring your arm back to your side, then swing it across your chest toward your other arm.

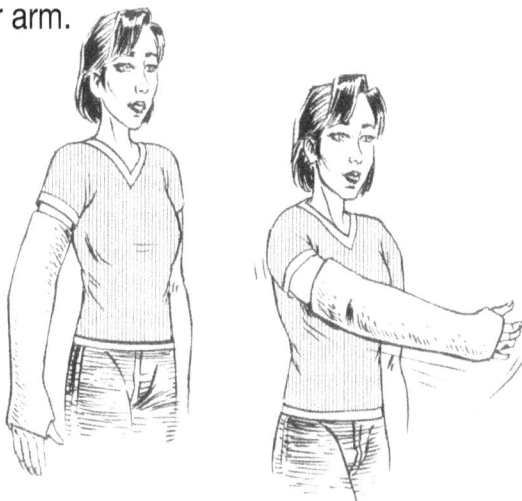

Exercising the hip

Sit in the middle of your bed with both legs extended directly in front of you. Move the casted leg slowly out to the far side as far as it will comfortably go. Then move it slowly back to its original position.

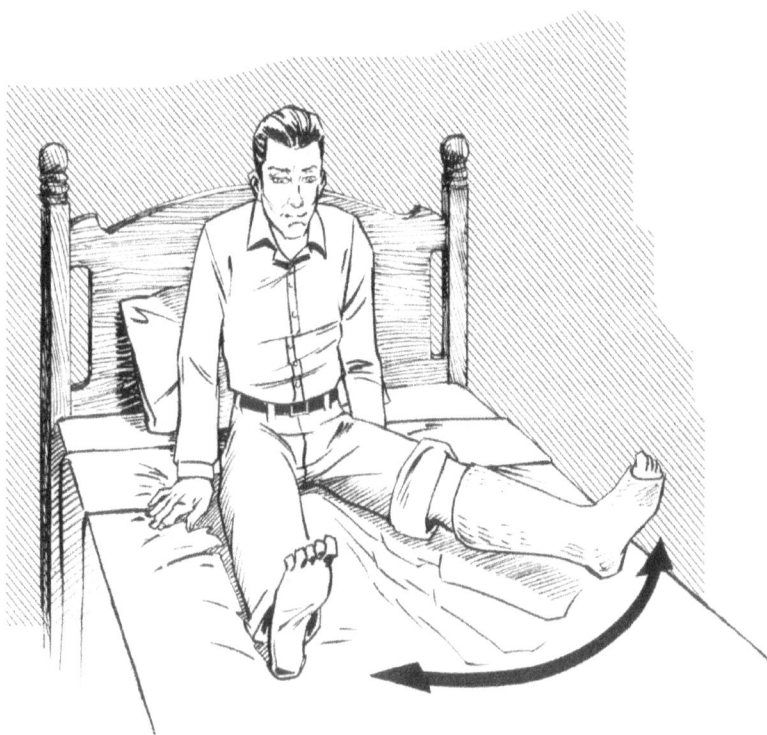

Exercising the ankle

Make a circle with your foot, first moving it clockwise, then counterclockwise. Next, stretch your foot so your toes reach back toward you and your heel juts away from you; then, reverse this position, so your toes stretch away from you.

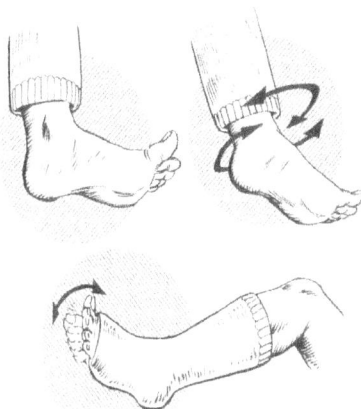

Exercising your toes

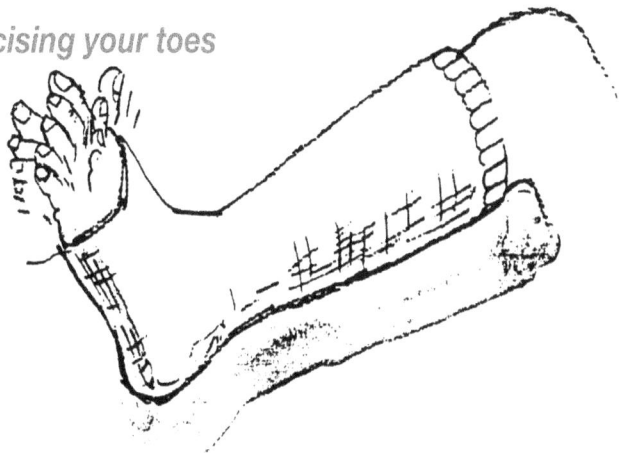

Wiggle your toes. If you have a short leg cast, bend and straighten the knee.

WHEN YOUR CAST IS REMOVED

C ast removal is fast and painless. The health care professional will probably remove the cast only when the broken bone has healed. However, the cast may have to be removed earlier if the break requires additional manipulation, if the cast becomes damaged, or becomes tight or loose, or if abnormal drainage signals a problem. You should never try to remove or trim the cast yourself.

Cutting the cast

Usually a specially designed saw will cut one side of the cast, then the other. This saw swiftly cuts through the stiff plaster.

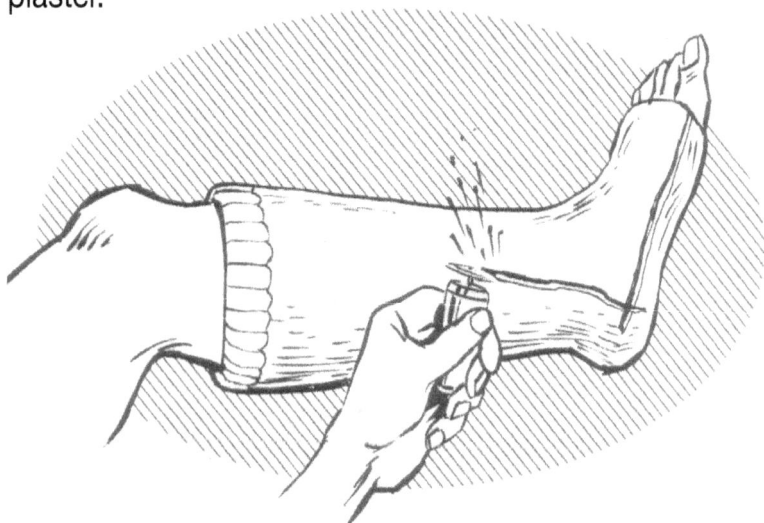

Opening the cast and removing the padding

After cutting the cast, the health care professional will open the cast pieces with a spreader. Then they will cut through the cast padding with special scissors, revealing a skin that may be covered with yellow or gray scales. This is due to the accumulation of dead skin, as well as oil from glands near the skin surface. The arm or leg will probably appear thinner and flabbier than the uncasted one, and it may ache and feel weak. This is due mostly to the muscle "wasting away" – the old adage "use it or lose it" especially applies to muscles. Don't worry, though, exercise and skin care will soon return the arm or leg to its normal condition.

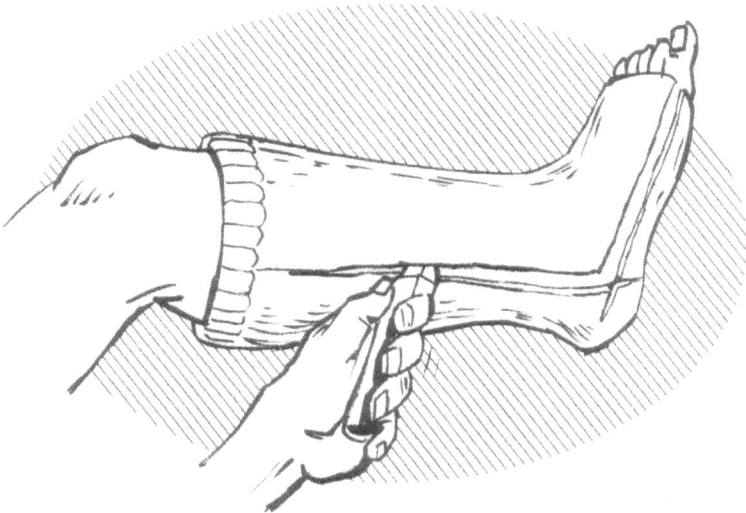

Cleaning the skin

After removing all the padding, the health care professional will wipe the arm or leg to remove debris. Wash with warm water and soap. If there is any skin damage, this should be treated appropriately.

When you return home, follow the cleaning instructions you have been given. Over time, all the accumulated dead skin will be loosened.

A skin cream may be recommended - follow the instructions.

Do not shave your limb immediately, wait 2-3 days, as a skin rash can occur, which can be severe at times.

EXERCISING AFTER YOUR CAST IS REMOVED

Your limb has been passive for many weeks, so you can expect your muscles to have lost their tone and some of their mass. Also, you will probably feel muscle stiffness and the joints will probably be less mobile. Do not despair; with time and the right exercises, everything can return to normal.

The benefits of exercise

We all know the feeling of well-being we get when we exercise; most people even have a better outlook on life. There are, however, dramatic medical benefits to exercising as well, namely:

- Improves the pumping action of the heart, with time, making it more efficient.
- Improves overall circulation to all parts of the body.
- Promotes well–being of the lungs, preventing possible future infections.
- Speeds up the gastrointestinal motion so that constipation can be prevented.
- Promotes urinary function by improving blood flow to the kidneys.

Types of exercise

Your physician, nurse, registered orthopedic technologist or physiotherapist should provide you with a range of specific exercises to help you get back to normal as quickly as possible. Follow the instructions and try to be self-disciplined in carrying out the exercises as often as recommended.

There are two types of exercises :

1. Range of Motion (ROM) exercises

These exercises involve moving your joints frequently and as progress occurs, the range of motion or how far you can extend your joints will improve. Coupled with this, your muscle strength will increase. It is vital that you follow the advice of your health care professional.

2. Stregthening exercises

Here, you do exercises against resistive forces which increase the muscle strengthening effect.

CARRYING OUT EXERCISES SAFELY

Always

• Follow your health care professional's advice exactly.
• Move slowly and gently to avoid injury.
• Stop exercising if you get tired.

Never

• Try to do exercises unless you have your health care professional's approval.
• Continue any exercise that causes pain. Stop immediately and check with your health care professional.
• Exercise to the point of exhaustion.

CAST CARE CHECKLIST

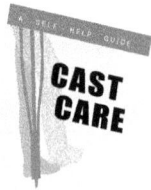

CAST CARE

Please read this book while waiting for your cast to dry or ask where you can obtain a copy if the clinic does not have supplies.

	Yes	No
Did the cast dry properly?	○	○
Do you know the type of cast material?	○	○
Do I know the cast care tips?	○	○
Do I understand MY situation about keeping my cast dry?	○	○
Have I considered the option of a waterproof cast, using a GORE® PROCEL® Cast Liner?	○	○
Do I know there are also external "cast protectors" that can keep my cast dry?	○	○
Do I know not to scratch inside my cast?	○	○
Do I know how to prevent swelling of limbs by elevation?	○	○
If applicable, do I know how to use crutches properly and safely?	○	○
Do I know the Warning Signs to phone the clinic for advice?	○	○
Did I read the booklet CAST CARE to ensure I understand what I have to do?	○	○

Hopefully you have answered yes to all of these questions.

Patient Name _____

Signature _____ Date _____

"Ask your clinic for a copy of this checklist"

www.medisript.net • Email: mediscript30@yahoo.ca • Toll Free 800 773 5088 • Fax: 800 639 3186

PROGRESS DIARY

Date of new cast _____

Date of cast removal _____

Special instructions _____

_____

_____

_____

_____

_____

_____

Problems, incidents, medical appointments, etc.

Week # ....

....

Week # ....

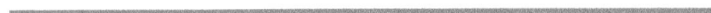

....

Week # ....

....

Week # ....

....

Week # ....

....

Week # ....

....

Week # ....

....

Week # ....

....

Week # ....

....

Week # ....

WARNING SIGNS
WHEN TO CALL YOUR DOCTOR
OR FRACTURE CLINIC

1. Increasing pain.

2. Pain that is not relieved by medication.

3. Excessive swelling that is not relieved by elevating the cast above the heart level for one hour.

4. Numbness, tingling or burning sensations in your toes or fingers.

5. A change in skin color above or below the cast.

6. A warm area or fresh stain on the cast.

7. A bad smell coming from within the cast.

8. If you drop an object onto the cast, or cast becomes damaged.

9. The cast becomes weakened, loose, broken or cracked.

10. The cast becomes too loose or too tight.

11. If the cast becomes wet.

12. Increasing pressure or painful rubbing inside the cast.

TO ORDER

PHONE: TOLL FREE   1 800 773 5088

FAX: TOLL FREE   1 800 639 3186

E-MAIL: mediscript30@yahoo.ca

Now Directly From Our Web-Site
www.mediscript.net

Name _____ Title _____

Address _____

_____

City _____ State/Prov. _____ Zip/Code _____

Tel. _____ Fax _____

Cell _____